All About
ORAL HYGIENE

By Laura Flynn R.N., B.N., M.B.A., in consultation with her nurse educator associates and physicians who assisted in contributing and editing.

ISBN No: 978 1 896616 73 5

© 2011, 2017 Mediscript Communications Inc.

The publisher, Mediscript Communications Inc., acknowledges the financial support of the Government of Canada through the Canadian Book Fund for our publishing activities.

Printed in Canada

www.mediscript.net

Book and Front Cover design by:
Brian Adamson, www.AdamsonGraphics.net

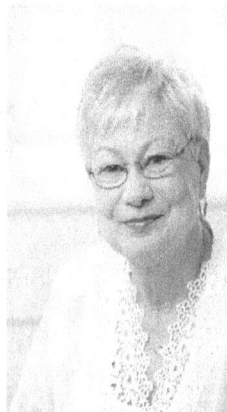

CONTENTS

INTRODUCTION

This book provides basic, non controversial and trusted information that can help a wide spectrum of readers.

The primary objective of the information is to help a person provide effective quality care to a loved one or someone in his or her care.

After reading this material you will have a better understanding of the importance of mouth care and its role in good overall hygiene. As well, you will be more prepared to assist the people in your care to a better quality of life.

All the information is reliable and was written by a group of eminent nurse educators who ensured the information complies with best practice guidelines and satisfies the various accreditation and regulatory bodies. Because there is so much unreliable information on the internet, you can be assured the "All About" publications are HON (Health On the Net) certified.

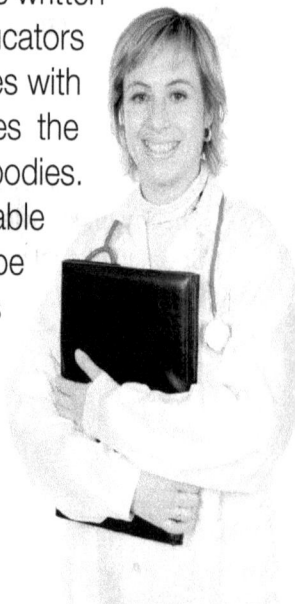

This book can be an invaluable aid to:

A caregiver caring for a relative or friend;
A health worker seeking a reference aid;
Any person involved in health care wishing to expand his or her knowledge.

AN IMPORTANT MESSAGE
FROM THE PUBLISHER

Each person's treatment, advice, medical aids, physical therapy and other approaches to health care are unique and highly dependant upon the diagnosis and overall assessment by the medical team.

We emphasize therefore that the information within this book is not a substitute for the advice and treatment from a health care professional.

This book provides generic information concerning the issues around oral hygiene and common sense, well-established mouth care practices for caregivers.

With all this in mind, the publishers and authors disclaim any responsibility for any adverse effects resulting directly or indirectly from the suggestions contained within this book or from any misunderstanding of the content on the part of the reader.

The following notices were found in various locations:

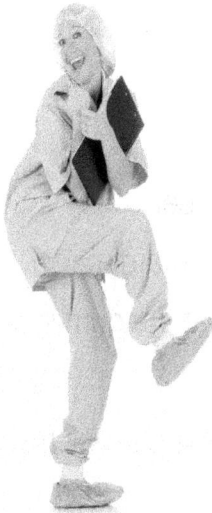

- **In a non-smoking area:**
  If we see you smoking, we will assume you are on fire and take appropriate action.

- **On the door of a maternity ward:**
  Push. Push. Push.

- **In a cemetery:**
  Persons are prohibited from picking flowers from any but their own graves.

- **On a highway:**
  When this sign is under water, this road is impassable.

HOW MUCH DO YOU KNOW?

It helps to figure out how much you know before starting. In this way you will have an idea as to the gaps in your knowledge prior to reading the content. Please circle to indicate the best answer. Remember, at this stage, you are not expected to know all the answers:

1. What is plaque?

A. A device for cleaning teeth

B. An invisible film that sticks to the teeth

C. A cleansing agent that prevents tooth decay

D. A hard deposit that can be seen at the gum line

2. Which group is most likely to have oral problems?

A. Young children

B. Teenagers

C. Middle-aged adults

D. The elderly

3. Why do many older people lose their teeth?

A. Periodontal disease

B. Side effect of medications

C. They opt to use false teeth

D. Side effect of a medical condition

4. How often should you assist people to brush their teeth?

A. At least once a day

B. At least twice a day

C. At least three times a day

D. After every meal

5. How often should you assist people to floss their teeth?

A. At least once a day

B. At least twice a day

C. At least three times a day

D. A minimum of four times a day

6. How long does it take for dental plaque to reoccur following removal?

A. 8 hours

B. 24 hours

C. 2 days

D. One week

7. How would you position an unconscious person to prevent aspiration when providing mouth care?

A. Sitting up in bed at a 90 degree angle

B. Sitting up slightly with an emesis dish nearby

C. On the side with the head of the bed lowered slightly

D. Sitting up at a 45 degree angle and head turned to the side

ANSWERS

1. B. Plaque is an invisible film that sticks to the enamel surface of the teeth and leads to tooth decay.

2. D. The elderly are at high risk for mouth problems.

3. A. Many older people lose their teeth due to periodontal disease.

4. B. Toothbrushing twice a day offers sufficient protection against tooth decay.

5. A. Flossing is usually done after brushing the teeth and at least once a day.

6. B. Dental plaque takes about 24 hours to reoccur once it has been thoroughly removed.

7. C. Position the person on the side with the head turned well to the side.

SOMETHING TO THINK ABOUT...

He who angers you conquers you.

Elizabeth Kenny

WHAT IS ORAL HYGIENE?

Oral hygiene (mouth care) involves cleansing of the mouth, gums, teeth and dentures. Oral hygiene is one aspect of care that is often neglected by care providers. Staff shortages and time constraints may make it difficult to provide the quality of care that is needed. Mouth care, however, is an important part of overall personal hygiene. When you assist people with their personal care, you must also ensure that they receive good oral hygiene. The information in this book will increase your knowledge about how to assist someone with oral hygiene.

Toothbrushing and flossing are important parts of good oral care. Plaque is an invisible film that sticks to the enamel surface of the teeth and leads to tooth decay. Toothbrushing helps loosen food particles, plaque, and bacteria. Flossing also helps remove plaque and prevent inflammation and infection.

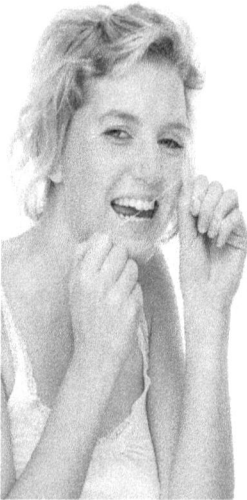

When plaque is not removed, it builds up over a period of time and turns into a hard substance called tartar. Tartar forms at the gum line and can lead to gum disease, the number one reason for tooth loss in adults. Tartar can be removed during cleaning by a dentist or dental hygienist.

Good oral hygiene has many benefits. It improves appetite, speech, general appearance, and dental health. Proper and regular oral care reduces mouth odors, gum disease, and cavities. The people in your care will feel better all over when their teeth are brushed and flossed.

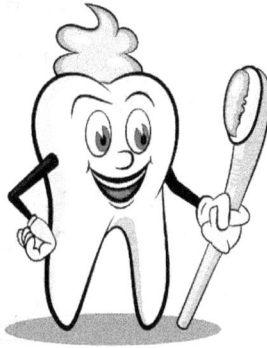

HOW OFTEN SHOULD YOU PROVIDE
ORAL HYGIENE?

Many healthcare workers are relieved to find out that toothbrushing twice a day and flossing once a day offer sufficient protection against cavities. That's because dental plaque takes about 24 hours to reoccur once it has been thoroughly removed. Assist the person with oral hygiene in the morning when you help him with his personal care and again at bedtime before he settles in for the night. (Some facilities may have policies that differ from these guidelines so find out about the rules in your workplace).

Check the care plan before you provide mouth care. Some people have special needs. The care plan will tell you the type of oral care the person needs and how often it should be done. For example, some people require mouth care as often as every 2 hours. If the care plan does not include information that you need, check with the person's doctor, dentist or health care professional.

KEY TERMS

Aspiration

Inhaling food into the lungs.

Autoimmune disease

One of a group of diseases in which the body forms antibodies against its own cells.

Chemotherapy

The use of chemicals to selectively destroy cancer cells.

Dementia

A brain disorder that worsens over time. Symptoms include memory loss as well as poor judgment and impulse control.

Dentures

Artificial teeth. Some people refer to dentures as "false teeth."

Flossing

Cleansing of tooth surfaces with dental floss or dental tape.

Human immunodeficiency virus (HIV)

A virus that attacks the body's immune system, making it difficult to fight disease.

Oral hygiene

Mouth care. It involves cleansing of the mouth, gums, teeth and dentures.

Periodontal disease

An inflammation of the tissues around the teeth.

Plaque

An invisible film that sticks to the enamel surface of the teeth and that leads to tooth decay.

Sponge swabs

Foam brushes. The foam replaces the bristles on a regular toothbrush. They are used to clean the oral cavity of people with painful, sensitive mouths or those who are unconscious.

Standard precautions

Guidelines that treat blood and other body fluids as if they were contagious, regardless of the source.

Stomatitis

Inflammation of the mouth.

Tartar

A hard deposit of plaque and bacteria that builds up over a period of time. It can be seen at the gum line.

RISK FACTORS FOR ORAL PROBLEMS

Many factors increase the risk of oral problems. These include lack of knowledge about mouth care, poor eating habits, and poor oral health practices. Illness or certain medications may cause dry mouth, bad breath, a bad taste in the mouth, a coated tongue, or sore gums. Other factors that affect oral health include:

- Poorly fitting dentures
- People who are not able to eat or drink (e.g. unconscious)
- People receiving oxygen therapy
- Mouth breathing
- A tube or airway in the mouth
- Exposure to alcohol or tobacco
- Suctioning

Certain groups are more likely to have oral problems. The elderly, for instance, are at high risk for mouth problems. Age-related changes can have a negative impact on oral health in several ways:

- Many older people lose their teeth due to **periodontal disease.** About half of the people in the United States who are 65 years or more wear dentures. Many others have no teeth at all.

- The surface of the teeth often wears down with age.

- Older people tend to have weak jaw muscles, making it more difficult to chew food. This change can lead to poor nutrition.

- The sense of taste decreases with age, contributing to poor nutrition.

- Saliva decreases, resulting in dry mouth. Older people are also more likely to take medications, which can lead to dry mouth. Certain products are available to reduce the symptoms of dry mouth. Extra fluids may help too.

- Many elderly people have diabetes, which is a risk factor for oral health problems. Older people with diabetes are at risk for all the oral health problems of aging along with others specific to their condition (inflammation, oral ulcers, and infection).

Other at-risk groups are those with certain types of **autoimmune disease** or renal (kidney) disease. About 40% of patients who receive **chemotherapy** for cancer develop **stomatitis**. Stomatitis can be very painful and can create difficulty with eating, drinking and talking.

Human immunodeficiency virus (HIV) attacks the body's immune system, making it difficult to fight disease. Common problems include dry mouth, mouth ulcers and sores, and swelling of the salivary glands. People who are very ill, unconscious or dying are also at increased risk for oral problems.

It's a mistake to assume that oral problems are inevitable. In most cases these problems can be prevented or successfully managed. Careful and regular oral hygiene, early reporting of unusual symptoms, regular dental visits, treatment with appropriate pain medication and antibiotics are all measures that can improve and resolve mouth problems.

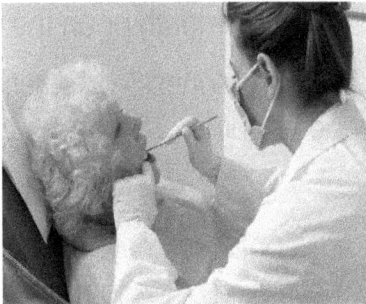

OBSERVING FOR PROBLEMS

As you provide oral care, you may become aware of problems. If you notice unusual symptoms or anything else that you are not sure of, call the person's health care professional. Early detection can often prevent small problems from developing into serious complications. Some of the signs and symptoms to report are:

- Bad breath
- Loose teeth
- Problems with swallowing
- Dry, cracked, or blistered lips
- Complaints of pain or discomfort
- Chipped, broken, or discolored teeth
- Chipped, broken, or poorly fitting dentures
- White patches in the mouth or on the tongue
- Bleeding, swelling, redness, or sores of the lips, mouth, tongue or gums

People who are confused may not be able to tell you when they have pain or discomfort. You will have to watch for signs of a possible problem. Pay close attention if the person begins grinding her teeth, hitting her jaw, or pulling on an ear.

Some people may refuse to eat, refuse to wear their dentures, or throw their dentures across the room. These could be signs of pain or discomfort and should be reported.

CONSIDER FOR A MOMENT ...

Have you observed other types of

behavior in response to oral pain and

discomfort? If so, what were they?

PROVIDING ORAL HYGIENE

Outlined below are procedures for common oral hygiene tasks. These include brushing and flossing the teeth, cleaning dentures, and mouth care for the unconscious person. The procedures are meant to be guidelines only. If you work for a healthcare agency, your workplace may have policies and procedures for you to follow. Remember too that every person is unique. Follow the person's care plan. Check for special instructions such as the need for pain relief medication before receiving mouth care. If you are unsure about something, ask the health care professional.

The first step in providing oral hygiene is to prepare the equipment you will need. Being organized enables you to provide care more efficiently and with fewer interruptions. Lay out any items you will need on paper towels on a work area within reach. Remember to ensure the person's privacy before beginning the procedure.

Inspecting someone's mouth and providing oral care brings you in contact with saliva, mucous membranes, and possibly blood. You can protect yourself and the person in your care against infection by using **standard precautions**. Standard precautions are guidelines that treat blood and other body fluids as if they were contagious, regardless of the source. Always wear gloves when giving oral hygiene.

CONSIDER FOR A MOMENT ...
What are the other
guidelines included in
standard precautions?

Never use your fingers to keep the person's mouth open when giving mouth care. Doing so will put you at risk of receiving a bite.

Carry out the procedure as outlined below. When you are finished, place the call bell within reach. Lower the bed to the lowest position (to decrease the risk of injury in the case of a fall) unless agency policy or the person's care plan directs otherwise.

Brushing the teeth

Some people will be able to gather their supplies and brush their teeth independently. Others may need your help just to set up the equipment. Still others will not be able to assist with the procedure at all. Changes can be made to standard toothbrushes to promote independence by improving the handgrip. An Occupational Therapist should be able to assist in this regard.

CONSIDER FOR A MOMENT ...
Are you caring for someone now who
could improve their grip on
their toothbrush?

Equipment Required

-Soft bristled toothbrush (or specialty toothbrush if recommended)

-Toothpaste or other oral cleaning agent

-Small bowl such as an emesis basin

-Straw if necessary

-Disposable gloves

-Towel and facecloth

-Mouthwash (optional)

-Paper towels

-Water

-Water-soluble lip lubricant

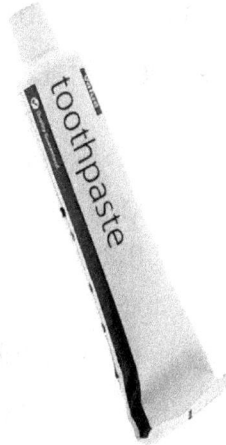

Procedure (Note: We'll assume here that you are caring for a female patient.)

1. Explain the procedure before you start.

2. Assist the person to a sitting position, next to a sink if possible. If providing care in bed, use the emesis basin. If the person cannot sit up, position the bed at a safe working level, and assist her to a side-lying position. Ensure her head is on a pillow.

3. Use a towel to keep her clothing dry.

4. Wash your hands.

5. Apply disposable gloves.

6. If her lips are dry, apply a lubricant in a thin layer to prevent drying and cracking. The lubricant should be a water-soluble one.

7. Wet the toothbrush with tepid water and apply toothpaste. The toothpaste should contain fluoride as fluoride helps prevent cavities. If she is someone who's at risk for mouth problems her dentist may order another type of cleaning agent.

8. If she is is able to brush her teeth independently, offer her the toothbrush and assist as required.

9. If she is not able to assist, begin to brush her teeth. Position the toothbrush at a 45-degree angle to her gum line.

10. Gently move the brush back and forth using short strokes.

11. Be sure to brush all the surfaces of the teeth. That would include the inner, outer, and chewing surfaces.

12. Gently brush the tongue if coated to remove bacteria and freshen the breath.

13. Offer her a drink of water to rinse the mouth. Use a straw if required. Hold the emesis basin if necessary so she can spit out the water.

14. If her lips are dry, apply a water-soluble lip lubricant again.

15. Offer mouthwash. Mouthwashes that contain alcohol can have a drying effect on oral tissue and irritate the mouth of someone with stomatitis. For these reasons, many healthcare agencies now use non-alcohol based mouthwashes.

16. Ensure she is as comfortable as possible.

17. Raise the siderails as per her care plan.

18. Clean the equipment and put away the supplies.

19. Remove your gloves and wash your hands.

20. Document the procedure in the appropriate place.

Flossing

Flossing is usually done after brushing the teeth and at least once a day. Flossing removes food particles and plaque from between the teeth. Assist the people in your care to floss independently if they can. You will need to floss for people who require help.

Equipment Required

Floss (or flossing device)

Disposable gloves

Water

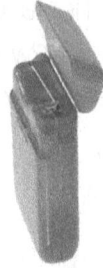

Procedure (Note: We'll assume here you're caring for a male patient.)

1. Wash your hands and apply disposable gloves.

2. Break off about 18 inches of floss. Waxed floss results in less fraying than unwaxed floss. Food particles, however, attach more easily to unwaxed floss.

3. Wind one end of the floss around the middle finger of each hand.

4. Hold the floss between your thumb and forefingers.

5. Move the floss between the teeth with a gentle rubbing motion.

6. Using up and down movements, gently rub the floss against the side of the teeth.

7. Repeat the procedure for all the teeth.

8. Don't forget to keep moving to a clean section of floss as you progress.

9. Once you are finished, offer him a glass of water to rinse the mouth.

10. Ensure he is as comfortable as possible.

11. Raise the siderails as per his care plan.

12. Clean the equipment and put away all of the items.

13. Remove your gloves and wash your hands.

14. Document the procedure in the appropriate place.

A number of flossing aids are available for use by patients or caregivers. These devices include floss wands, floss piks, special brushes, and sticks. Many older people have never gotten into the habit of flossing. They may refuse to floss their teeth or to have you do it for them. You must respect their wishes. Let your supervisor or healthcare professional know that they would prefer not to have their teeth flossed.

CLEANING DENTURES

If you are caring for an elderly person, it is quite likely that he or she will have dentures (artificial teeth). Dentures may consist of an upper or lower plate or both. Keep in mind that dentures are very expensive items. Many people do not have extra money to replace missing or damaged dentures. Do all you can to ensure the dentures are properly cared for.

Encourage the people in your care to wear their dentures. People who do not wear their dentures are at risk of shrinkage of the gums and further tooth loss. Like natural teeth, artificial dentures need to be cleaned regularly. They should be cleaned at least once a day. Use only recommended cleaning agents. Otherwise you may damage the dentures.

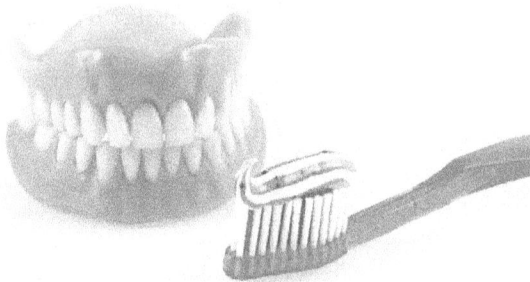

Handle dentures with extreme care. They can easily slip out of your hands and break. They can crack or chip even if they fall in the sink. Ensure that you use gauze or a tissue to remove them from the person's mouth. The gauze or tissue will improve your grip on the dentures. Place a washcloth (or small towel) in the sink when you are cleaning dentures. Never use hot water for cleaning as it can change the shape of the dentures.

Dentures should be removed at night. This helps to give the gums a rest and prevent a buildup of bacteria. When not in use, dentures should be placed in cool water in a denture cup. Clearly label the cup so that your patient's dentures are not mistaken for someone else's. As well, most facilities have denture-marking kits on hand for labeling of dentures. Labeling is the best way to ensure that someone's dentures do not wind up in someone else's mouth.

Some people will be independent in caring for their dentures, while others will need some assistance from you. Still others will not be able to assist with the procedure at all. To promote independence, encourage people to help with denture care to the extent that they are able.

Equipment Required

Denture cup

Small bowl such as an emesis basin

Soft-bristled toothbrush or denture brush

Toothpaste or other recommended cleaning agent

Denture cleaner

Towel

Washcloth (or small towel)

Tissue or gauze

Disposable gloves

Mouthwash

Paper towels

Cup of cool water

Procedure (Note: We will assume here that the person in your care is a woman.)

1. Explain the procedure before you begin.

2. Assist her to a sitting position.

3. Use a towel to keep her clothing dry.

4. Wash your hands.

5. Put on disposable gloves.

6. Ask her to remove her dentures and place them in the basin. If she is unable to do so, remove the dentures. Using a tissue or gauze, grasp the top dentures at the front teeth with your thumb and forefinger. Move the denture up and down gently to break the suction. Remove the bottom denture by lifting upwards while turning slightly to one side. Place the dentures in the denture cup. Carefully take them to the sink.

7. Place a washcloth (or small towel) in the sink to help prevent the dentures from breaking if you drop them.

8. Under tepid running water, rinse the dentures. Instructions on some cleaning agents are to use cool or warm water.

9. Holding the dentures in the palm of your hand, use the brush and scrub them with toothpaste or other cleaning agent. Rinse well.

10. If the dentures are stained, they can be soaked in a commercial denture cleaner. Follow the directions on the package if you do so. Dentures with metal parts should not be soaked overnight to prevent wearing away of the metal.

11. Offer her a glass of water or mouthwash so she can rinse her mouth.

12. Ensure the dentures are well rinsed before they are placed back into her mouth.

13. Ensure she is as comfortable as possible.

14. Raise the siderails as per her care plan.

15. Clean the equipment and put away the supplies.

16. Remove your gloves and wash your hands.

17. Document the procedure in the appropriate place.

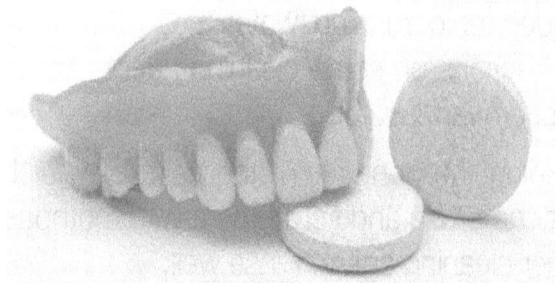

MOUTH CARE FOR THE
UNCONSCIOUS PERSON

People who are unconscious cannot tell you if they feel pain or discomfort. They usually cannot swallow. They often breathe through the mouth and receive oxygen, factors which cause mouth dryness and increase the risk of infection. Because of all these special challenges, unconscious people require mouth care at least every two hours.

The procedure below uses **sponge swabs** for mouth care of unconscious people. Sponge swabs are also useful for people with painful or sensitive mouths. They do not clean as well as toothbrushes, however, and should be used in moderation. Special mouthwashes are sometimes prescribed to increase the effectiveness of the sponge swabs.

When using a sponge swab, ensure that the sponge pad is tightly attached to the stick. If not, it may dislodge and cause choking. Avoid using sponge swabs on someone who is combative due to the risk that he or she may bite off the sponge and choke on it.

Unconscious people are at risk for choking and aspiration. **Aspiration** means inhaling fluid into the lungs. People who aspirate can become ill with pneumonia. To prevent aspiration, position the unconscious person properly before you begin mouth care. Even with proper positioning, oral suctioning may be needed. Some healthcare facilities have two staff (one of whom would be a registered nurse) assist with providing mouth care for an unconscious client – one person uses the suction while the other staff member provides the mouth care.

Many facilities routinely use soft bristled toothbrushes rather than sponge swabs for oral care of unconscious clients. If you do use a toothbrush, brush gently to avoid harming the gums. Rinse gently with small amounts (about 10 ml. of water) after brushing. A syringe (without the needle) can be used to gently inject the water into each side of the mouth. Special toothbrushes that connect directly to a wall suction are also available. Refer to the person's care plan and check with the healthcare professional before providing mouth care to an unconscious person.

Equipment

Oral cleaning agent

Sponge swabs

Tongue blades, tape, and gauze

Cup of cool water

Towel

Small bowl such as an emesis basin

Disposable gloves

Paper towels

Water-soluble lip lubricant

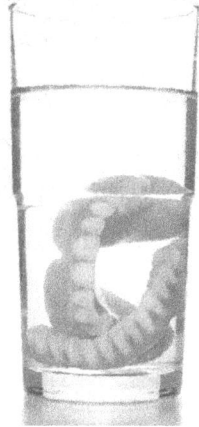

Procedure (Note: We'll assume here that the unconscious person is a man.)

1. Explain the procedure before you begin. **Many unconscious people are able to hear even though they cannot speak or respond to what you are saying.** Talk to the person throughout the entire procedure. Explain what you plan to do each step of the way.

2. Position the bed at a safe working level.

3. Place a towel under his chin.

4. Wash your hands.

5. Apply disposable gloves.

6. If his lips are dry, apply a thin layer of water-soluble lip lubricant before starting brushing.

7. Position him on the side with his head turned well to the side. Lower the head of the bed slightly. This will allow any excess liquid to flow out of his mouth and away from his throat.

8. Position all equipment within easy reach to ensure you do not have to leave him during the procedure.

9. Place the emesis basin under his chin to collect any fluid that comes from the mouth.

10. Insert the mouth prop quickly but gently between his teeth. The mouth prop provides an open area for you to work (See the section Using a Mouth Prop).

11. You are now ready to begin cleansing the mouth. Use sponge swabs moistened with the oral cleaning agent. The person you are caring for may be ordered a specific cleaning agent on the care plan.

12. Do not use a lot of fluid on the sponge swab for cleaning or rinsing so as to avoid the risk of aspiration.

13. Clean the chewing and inner surfaces of the teeth first. Then continue to clean the outer

surfaces of the teeth. The roof of the mouth, inside of the cheeks, and the lips should be swabbed to remove secretions and crusts. The tongue should be gently swabbed. Take caution not to stimulate the gag reflex as you do so.

14. To rinse the mouth, moisten a clean sponge swab with water and swab the mouth. Repeat the rinse several times.

15. Dry his face and mouth with a towel.

16. If his lips are dry, apply water-soluble lip lubricant again.

17. Remove the towel.

18. Ensure he is as comfortable as possible.

19. Raise the siderails as per his care plan.

20. Clean the equipment and put away the supplies.

21. Remove your gloves and wash your hands.

22. Document the procedure in the appropriate place.

Avoid using lemon and glycerine swabs when giving mouth care to unconscious people. These swabs have a drying effect on the mucous membranes and can also erode tooth enamel. Oral Balance mouth moisturizing gel is an acceptable substitute used in some facilities.

Using a mouth prop

Mouth props may be used for people who are unable, due to illness, aging, or because they are unconscious, to hold their mouth open for mouth care. A mouth prop can be used to separate the upper and lower teeth. To make a mouth prop, wrap several 2x2 gauze squares around one half of two tongue blades and then tape it in place. Use more tongue blades if you need a wider opening.

When using a mouth prop, place the prop on one side of the mouth and then thoroughly clean the other side. Move the mouth prop and repeat. A rolled-up facecloth placed between the teeth works well, too. Leave the mouth prop in for brief periods, giving spells of rest in between. For the person who may bite down on the mouth prop, omit the gauze. Instead tape together as many tongue blades as you will need, depending on the size of the opening you require.

THE PERSON WITH DEMENTIA

People with **dementia** may not always cooperate with procedures such as toothbrushing. Nevertheless, every effort should be made to carry out mouth care twice a day even if only for a few seconds each time. Some suggestions that may help are:

- Attempt oral care when the person is rested and comfortable. If unsuccessful at first, try later.

- Try a collis curve toothbrush (if back teeth are present). A collis curve toothbrush cleans three sides of the teeth at once and can speed up the cleaning process for people with a limited attention span.

- Ask a partner to assist with providing oral care if the person is confused and combative.

- Don't use sponge swabs on confused people who may resist care as they may bite off a piece and choke.

- Keep mouth care products out of reach of confused people.

Oral products containing chlorhexidine are sometimes used in addition to toothbrushing. Chlorhexidine is a chemical that helps reduce the formation of plaque. Products that contain chlorhexidine should be used upon the advice of a professional. A common side effect is staining of the teeth.

CONSIDER FOR A MOMENT ...
Based upon any previous
experience you may have caring
for people with dementia,
can you add to this
list of suggestions?

CASE EXAMPLE

You have just begun to care for Mrs. Casey, an 83-year-old woman who is confused and has a history of heart disease. Mrs. Casey lives at home with her daughter and son-in-law. She wanders around the house all day but sleeps well at night. The daughter is concerned because, although her mother has always had a healthy appetite, she is presently eating poorly. Mrs. Casey has also begun grinding her teeth.

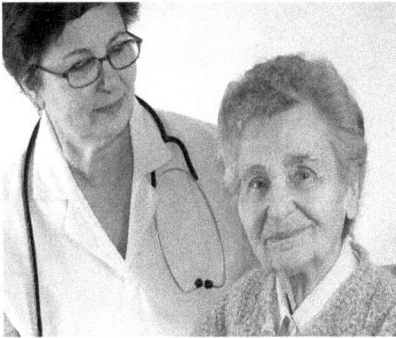

What risk factors for oral problems are present in this situation?

What symptoms of possible oral problems are present?

What can you do to help Mrs. Casey in this situation?

YOUR ANSWERS TO CASE EXAMPLE

SUGGESTED ANSWERS TO CASE EXAMPLE

What risk factors for oral problems are present in this situation?

A risk factor for oral problems present in this situation is advanced age (Mrs. Casey is eighty-three years old). As Mrs. Casey is confused, she is probably not following good oral care habits such as brushing and flossing. Poor oral practices, therefore, also put Mrs. Casey at risk for oral problems.

What symptoms of possible oral problems are present?

Mrs. Casey's eating habits have changed. She currently eats very little food each day. As well, she has begun grinding her teeth. Both of these changes can indicate oral pain or discomfort.

What can you do to help Mrs. Casey in this situation?

Mrs. Casey may need to be seen by a dentist. Inform your supervisor about the tooth grinding and the change in this person's appetite. Report any other unusual signs (refer to the section "Observing for Problems").

CONCLUSION

Good oral hygiene is an important part of overall hygiene for the person in your care. Providing good oral care to someone doesn't need to be a time-consuming and difficult task. It does, however, require planning and a certain level of skill on the caregiver's part. Good oral hygiene, provided on a regular basis, can help prevent serious mouth problems.

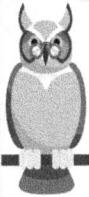

CHECK YOUR KNOWLEDGE

1. What are the risk factors for oral problems?

2. What are the signs of potential oral problems?

3. How would you position an unconscious person prior to providing mouth care?

4. Identify three ways that caregivers can help safeguard dentures from loss or damage.

5. Name three important points to keep in mind when brushing someone's teeth.

SPECIALTY DENTAL PRODUCT SUPPLIERS

The following websites will be helpful to you if you wish to find out more about the collis toothbrush, suction toothbrush or a variety of other products used to enhance mouth care:

Collis Curve Toothbrushes
www.colliscurve.com
1-800-298-4848 (US)

Plak-Vac Oral Suction Toothbrush
www.trademarkmedical.com
1-800-323-2220 (US)

Biotene Dry Mouth Products
www.biotene.net
1-800-922-5856 (US)
1-800-667-3770 (Canada)

Sage Products Inc.
www.sageproducts.com
1-800-323-2220 (US)

Germiphene
Provides products that contain chlorhexidine
www.germiphene.com
1-800-265-9931 (Canada)

Specialized Care Company
www.specializedcare.com
1-800-722-7375 (US)

TEST YOURSELF

Please circle to indicate the best answer:

1. Why would you use a tissue or gauze when handling dentures?

A. To decrease the risk of infection

B. To improve your grip on the dentures

C. To prevent tight gripping that could lead to cracks

D. To prevent them from breaking in case you drop them

2. How would you advise someone in your care regarding use of her dentures at night?

A. Wear them always, even at night

B. Store in a dry denture cup

C. Store in hot water in a denture cup

D. Store in cool water in a denture cup

3. How should you position the toothbrush while brushing someone's teeth?

A. 30 degree angle to the gum line

B. 45 degree angle to the gum line

C. 60 degree angle to the gum line

D. 90 degree angle to the gum line

4. While planning oral care, you are informed that this person tends to bite down on the mouth prop. What should you do?

A. Ignore the behaviour

B. Do not use a mouth prop

C. Use more gauze padding

D. Omit the gauze and use several taped blades instead

5. Which substance has a possible side effect of staining of the teeth?

A. Lemon and glycerine swabs

B. Hydrogen peroxide

C. Oral balance mouth moisturizing gel

D. A mouth rinse containing chlorhexidine

6. What are standard precautions?

A. Wearing gloves when caring for anyone

B. Guidelines that treat blood and body fluids as if they were contagious

C. Precautions you take only when you know the person has an infection

D. Precautions you take to prevent the onset of oral hygiene problems

7. How should you react to the person who does not wish to floss his teeth?

A. Tell him that flossing is not important anyway

B. Get a coworker to hold him down as you floss the teeth

C. Inform the person that he will lose all his teeth if he doesn't floss

D. Respect his wishes and let the healthcare professional know about the refusal

ANSWERS

1. B. Using gauze or tissue will improve your grip on the dentures.

2. D. When not in use, dentures should be placed in cool water in a denture cup.

3. B. Position the toothbrush at a 45-degree angle to the person's gum line.

4. D. For the person who may bite down on the mouth prop, omit the gauze. Instead tape together as many tongue blades as you will need, depending on the size of the opening you require.

5. D. Products that contain chlorhexidine should be used upon the advice of a professional. A common side effect is staining of the teeth.

6. B. Standard precautions are guidelines that treat blood and other body fluids as if they were contagious, regardless of the source.

7. D. You must respect his wishes. Let your supervisor or the healthcare professional know that this person would prefer not to have his teeth flossed.

REFERENCES

American Dental Association (ADA). (2004). Cleaning your teeth and gums (Oral Hygiene). Retrieved August 20, 2004, from: http://www.ada.org/public/topics/cleaning_faq.asp

Anderson, D. (Ed.). (2002). Mosby's medical, nursing, & allied health dictionary (6th ed.). St. Louis, MO: Mosby.

Brown, C. & Yoder, L. (2002). Stomatitis: An overview: Protecting the oral cavity during cancer treatment. American Journal of Nursing, 102 (4), 20-23.

Clift, A. (2004). Revising a nursing mouth care policy. Canadian Journal of Dental Hygiene (CJDH), 38 (5), 226-230.

Dahlin, C. (2004). Oral complications at the end of life. American Journal of Nursing, 104 (7), 40-47.

Kozier, B., Berman, A., Burke, K., Bouchal, D., & Hirst, S. (2004). Fundamentals of

Nursing. The Nature of Nursing Practice in Canada (First Canadian Edition). Toronto, ON: Prentice-Hall.

Lueckenotte, A. (2000). Gerontologic nursing (2nd ed.). St. Louis, MO: Mosby.

Potter, P., &, Perry, A.G. (2004). Basic nursing essentials for practice (5th ed.). St. Louis, MO: Mosby.

Sage Products. (2003). Supplement: Oral care update: From prevention to treatment. Nursing Management, 34 (5), 1-11.

Sorrentino, S. (2004). Mosby's Canadian textbook for the support worker. Toronto, ON: Mosby.

www.ingramcontent.com/pod-product-compliance
Lightning Source LLC
Chambersburg PA
CBHW060643280326
41933CB00012B/2138